LUNG CANCER (METASTATIC)

A survival guide for patients

Dr. Bhratri Bhushan
MBBS, MD, DM

therapeutic range. To the maximum extent permitted under applicable law, no responsibility is assumed by the publisher for any injury and/or damage to persons or property as a matter of products liability, negligence law or otherwise, or from any reference to or use by any person of this work.

Dedicated to my father Dr. Bharat Bhushan

CONTENTS

PREFACE

Lung cancer is one of the most common cancers, it is also the leading cause of cancer related mortality. With the advent of new diagnostic and therapeutic modalities, the management landscape of metastatic lung cancer has dramatically changed, especially so in the past decade.

In this book, together we will explore the subject of metastatic lung cancer. This will help you understand the disease better. It is overwhelming to know that either you or your loved one has been diagnosed with metastatic lung cancer and it may sound unrealistic that at this trying time you should pick up a book and understand the disease biology and management strategies but believe me, it is important. Today all of the decision making in medicine, especially in oncology, is "shared" decision making. What it means is that the team treating you is just one part of the decision making process, the other part is you and your family. An informed decision is a good decision and to make an informed decision, you must have reasonably enough knowledge of the subject.

The goal of this book is in no way to be an all encompassing, comprehensive reference for all of your questions; but to provide you all of the useful information, without unnecessarily burdening you with confusing facts and figures.

I have constructed this book in an interactive format, i.e., questions and answers. Most of these question I have picked up by my daily encounters with patients and their families and some I have constructed myself to bridge the gaps between the topics.

I hope you will find this book helpful. I wish you and your loved ones long, healthy and prosperous lives.

If you have any queries or suggestions, please contact me at bhratri@gmail.com

Q&AS

Q1. What is lung cancer?

Answer: many types of abnormal growths may be seen in the lungs, not all of them are cancers. Nowadays "screening" for lung cancers is recommended in some healthy people, if they fulfil certain criteria. Many times abnormal growths may be seen in lungs but most of the times they come out to be benign (non cancerous) on further evaluation.

Lung cancers are cancers that are primarily derived from the cells of lungs themselves. Remember that cancers from other areas of body may also spread to the lungs, but they will not be classified as lung cancers. For example, if a lung mass(es) is present in a patient with proven breast cancer, it will be known as metastatic breast cancer. In some instances, however, two cancers may occur simultaneously but that's very rare.

Q2. Are all lung cancers the same?

Answer: No. "Lung cancer" is not just one disease, it is a very broad term which encompasses very different biologic types of cancers affecting lungs.

There are following two broad types of lung cancers:

1. Non-small cell lung cancer
2. Small cell lung cancer

Non-small cell lung cancer (NSCLC) is the most common type of lung cancer. It is further divided into following types:

1. Squamous cell lung caner
2. Non-squamous cell lung cancer

Non-squamous cell NSCLC is the most common type of lung cancer. There are many types of it as well:

1. Adenocarcinoma (most common)
2. Large cell carcinoma
3. Other rare types

There are different properties of the cancers within the same type as well. For example, a patient having adenocarcinoma may or may not have certain mutations like EGFR, ALK, ROS1, BRAF etc. Lung cancers may be positive or negative for PD-L1. We will discuss these topics later on in this book.

So as we can clearly see from our discussion, lung cancer is not a single disease entity. There are many different varieties of lung cancers, the treatment plans for which may be very different. This classification of lung cancers also helps in prognostication.

Q3. Why have I developed lung cancer?

Answer: there are many risk factors, which predispose a person to develop lung cancer. Cigarette smoking is the most important risk factor. It is a modifiable risk factor.

That being said, it is not the only risk factor. Many times lung cancer occurs in patients who have never smoked or who had quit a long time ago.

Second hand smoke is another important risk factor. If someone in your proximity is smoking a cigarette and you inhale that smoke, it is known as second hand smoke.

There are many other causative agents like radon gas, heavy metals, asbestos et cetera. Sometimes lung cancer may run in families but such cases are rare.

Q4. I smoke cigarettes (or used to smoke), what are my chances of developing lung cancer?

Answer: this is common knowledge that cigarette smoking causes many types of cancers, one of which is lung cancer.

Remember that cigarette smoking is "risk" factor not only for lung cancer but many other types of cancers. On top of that, smoking is associated with increased incidence of heart diseases, lung diseases etc. So, lung cancer is not the only thing you have to consider.

There are mathematical models that are available on the web for calculation of your risk. These models take you age, age when you started to smoke, the number of cigarettes you smoke every day et cetera into account. If you want to take my advice, it will be this: no amount of cigarette smoking is "safe". Even if you smoke one cigarette a day, you are at risk. It is my sincere advice to you that you must completely stop smoking. There are better things to do in life than smoking a burning stick.

It is very important to note here that smoking cessation is strongly advised even after developing cancer. In fact, it will be the first advice that you will receive upon visiting your oncologist. Continuing to smoke after developing lung cancer has shown to decrease lifespan further, to diminish the effect of drugs and to increase the toxicities of treatment. Continuing to smoke may also lead to development of new cancers.

Q5. I smoke e-cigarettes, what about their impact on my chances of getting lung cancer?

Answer: it's too early to say. Electronic cigarettes, e-cigarettes or vaping are relatively new habits and while they appear safer compared with conventional cigarettes, further studies are needed to assess the risks they may pose. For the time being, the stand of international cancer organisations on the impact of e-cigarettes on lung cancer risk is unclear.

Q6. I know many people who have smoked through-out their lives and now they are in their eighties or nineties without any health problems whatsoever. What do you have to say about that?

Answer: as we have already discussed, cigarette smoking is a "risk factor", not a certainty factor. Cigarette smoking causes mutations in cells of the lungs, which accumulate over many decades before manifesting as cancer. The development of lung cancer depends on your genetics and other factors.

Think of it this way, if you always cross the road with eyes closed, will you always have an accident? And if you are always vigilant while crossing the road, will you never have an accident? All that we have in our power is to do our best in life, the rest is up to luck and risk.

Q7. My doctor says I have stage IV lung cancer, what does it mean?

Answer: please remember that stage IV lung cancer is not a single disease entity. Each patient with stage IV lung cancer is different.

Stage IV lung cancer is also known as metastatic lung cancer. When lung cancer is no longer confined to a lung and its associated lymph nodes and spreads beyond to involve other organs, it is said to have metastasised.

Following are some examples of metastatic lung cancer:
1. Lung cancer that causes pleural effusion (fluid surrounding the lung) or pericardial effusion (fluid surrounding the heart). Remember that sometimes, formation of such fluid may not be due to cancer. If you have pleural or pericardial effusion, you doctor will test its sample for presence of cancer cells and only after the confirmation of presence of cancer cells in the fluid can the lung cancer be labelled metastatic.
2. Lung cancer that has spread to the other lung. These are known as lung to lung metastases. Sometimes there may be two different cancers affecting the two lungs separately but it's a rare phenomenon.
3. Lung cancer that has spread to other organs. Lung cancer tends to spread to

bones, liver, adrenal glands and brain. Less frequently, it may spread to other organs as well. For example if the lung cancer has spread to the backbones, it will be considered metastatic. It may not be necessary to prove the presence of cancer cells in the organs to which it has spread and the diagnosis in such cases is based on the findings of studies like CT scans etc.

Q8. How does lung cancer spread?

Answer: lung cancer starts in some part of the lung, it then increases in size and affects more and more parts of that lung. It spreads outside of the lungs by two main routes: lymph and blood.

You may hear statements like "your lung cancer has spread to lymph nodes". There are lymph nodes in our body, which are part of the lymphatic system. They are part of our immune system. Lung cancer cells spread to the lymph nodes frequently. If this happens then it doesn't mean that it has metastasised. There are specific lymph nodes which are anatomically related to lungs, their involvement confers an advanced stage. If the lung cancer spreads to lymph nodes that are not related to lungs, then it is considered metastatic. For example if the cancer is in the right lung and it spreads to the supra-clavicular lymph node on the right side (which is a lymph node group situated above the collar bone), it is considered N3 nodal involvement and if there are no other sites of spread, it will be considered stage III. If on the other hand, the same lung cancer spreads to the nodes in the upper part of neck, it will be considered stage IV (metastatic).

Spread to more distant organs, like brain, adrenal glands and liver, occurs more commonly through the blood. If lung cancer is left untreated, it eventually becomes metastatic.

Q9. My primary care physician has suspicions that I may have metastatic lung cancer. What can I expect when I visit my oncologist for the first time?

Answer: lung cancer is often diagnosed in the late stages, and even when it appears to be localised on initial examinations, it may come out to be metastatic on further studies.

Your oncologist will perform the following tests for evaluation of lung cancer:

1. He will obtain your medical history. Your smoking habits and other details will also be obtained in detail.
2. He will record routine parameters like heart rate, blood pressure, breathing rate and temperature.
3. He will touch different areas of your body and listen to various sounds by stethoscope.
4. He will order blood tests.
5. He will order imaging tests. The imaging tests may include the following, as needed:
    1. CT scan of chest and abdomen.
    2. MRI of brain.
    3. PET-CT scan.
6. He will order a biopsy.
7. Depending on the results of the biopsy, further tests will be done:
    1. Immunohistochemistry testing
    2. Driver mutation testing etc.

Other tests like lung function tests, heart function tests etc. may be ordered. If you are suffering from any other diseases, their present status will also be evaluated.

Q10. Which is the best test for detecting metastatic lung cancer?

Answer: this is a very good question and it deserves thorough explanation.

Nowadays a PET-CT scan is performed in almost all patients suspected of having metastatic lung cancer. A PET-CT scan is a special type of imaging technique. It not only shows structural details of organs, but it also (in most cases) shows cancers as "hot" areas. To compare it with a CT scan, if there is a growth present in the lung, the CT scan will show the growth but it will not tell us about the physiology of the growth. On the other hand, a PET-CT scan uses a chemical "18-FDG" (there are other chemicals as well). The chemical is preferentially taken up by cancer cells, which then show increased uptake on PET scan and appear as "hot" areas.

But remember that if your PET-CT scan shows such abnormalities, they may not necessarily be due to cancer. There are many other diseases which may appear as hot areas on a PET-CT, for example infections and granulomatous diseases. Sometimes, the overall clinical scenario is such that there is no need to prove all the abnormalities that exist on a PET-CT and they may by considered cancerous. But in most circumstances, your doctor will obtain a sample from an area that appear abnormal on PET-CT and that sample will then undergo a pathologic examination to confirm the presence of cancer.

A point to remember is that PET-CT scan may miss the cancer present in brain. Brain is a common site of spread of lung cancer, and thus it is important to obtain a brain MRI in every patient with suspected metastatic lung cancer.

In summary, in my opinion the best combination of tests for initial evaluation of metastatic lung cancer is a PET-CT scan and an MRI of brain. You may have certain conditions which may make you unfit to undergo either or both of these tests. In that case, other tests like plain CT scans, ultrasound etc. are used.

Q11. My doctor says that based on my PET-CT scan (or CT scan) reports, she suspects I may have metastatic lung cancer. Do I have to undergo biopsy now? Can treatment be started without a biopsy? I am afraid of undergoing a biopsy.

Answer: you must understand this clearly: every patient with lung cancer has to undergo a biopsy. A biopsy is a very very safe procedure. Complications occur in a small minority of patients undergoing biopsy and even these complications are almost never serious.

The site from which a biopsy should be obtained is not similar in all the patients. Choosing the site form which to obtain a biopsy is crucial for many reasons. Your doctor will be the best judge in this matter. There are a few principles that doctors usually follow:

1.   Usually the site of biopsy is one which is the easiest to access and potentially least harmful for the patient.
2.   Usually the site of biopsy is one which will confer the highest stage, if found to be involved by cancer.
3.   The site of biopsy must be such that an adequate sample can be obtained for further testing.

Biopsies in cases of suspected metastatic lung cancer can be of following types:

1.   If you have fluid surrounding your lungs or heart, you doctor may choose to remove part of that fluid for examination. When part of the fluid surrounding lungs is removed, it is known as thoracentesis. When part of fluid surrounding heart is removed, it is known as peri-

cardiocentesis. These fluids are removed with the help of needles that are carefully guided by help of ultrasound or CT scans, through your skin into the fluid. After these fluids are removed, they are checked for presence of cancer cells under a microscope and further tests can be done on special "cell blocks" prepared from these fluids.

2. If you have an apparently affected, accessible and adequately sized supraclavicular node present, your doctor may choose to perform a core biopsy of it.

3. If your cancer is such that the only feasible site for obtaining a biopsy is the lung mass, then the method chosen will depend on the site of the tumor.

    1. Some lung tumors can be biopsied by a needle that pierces your skin and goes into the tumor, this technique is known as transthoracic needle aspiration/biopsy.

    2. Some lung tumor are best biopsied with a help of endoscopy. One commonly used method is EUS (endoscopic ultrasound) guided biopsy, other methods like bronchoscopy, endobronchial ultrasound etc. may also be used. In these endoscopic methods, a tube is inserted through your throat

and it travels through your wind-pipe to your lungs and special needles are there inside these tubes that are used for biopsy.

4.   Sometimes, the tumor can not be accessed by the above mentioned techniques. In these cases surgery may need to be done. Surgery may be minimally invasive or open surgery.

There are many myths surrounding a biopsy. Few examples of these myths are:
1.   A biopsy is very painful.
2.   A biopsy can kill me.
3.   A biopsy can spread cancer.
4.   A biopsy can activate cancer.
5.   A biopsy will inflame cancer.

These myths are unfounded and downright misleading. Please be sure that none of these is true. Biopsies are one the safest procedures and the information obtained from a biopsy forms the basis of your treatment.

Q12. I have undergone a biopsy for my suspected metastatic lung cancer. What tests will now be required before starting treatment?

Answer: metastatic cancer is mainly treated with medicines. Surgery may be required for certain symptoms but its role in the overall treatment is very limited. Radiation therapy may be needed, but it's also not the primary modality for the treatment of metastatic lung cancer.

In the past, there were very few options available for treatment of metastatic lung cancer. Nowadays there are many drugs available. Not any drug can be used in every patient of metastatic lung cancer, the proper selection of the drugs is guided by various tests.

The biopsy sample will be subjected to the following tests, which are described in detail below:
1. Histopathologic examination: this examination is done with the help of a microscope. It will reveal the "histology" of lung cancer. Further details of histologic types of metastatic lung cancer are provided in the question number 2.
2. Sometimes microscopy alone is not sufficient for histologic classification of the cancer. In such cases, immunohistochemistry examination is done. In this examination, special dyes are used to stain cancer cells, which are studied with the help

of a microscope.

3. Histologically lung cancer may be of small cell type or non-small cell type. If lung cancer is of small cell type, further evaluation is not usually necessary and treatment for metastatic small cell lung cancer is started.

4. If lung cancer is of non-small cell type. It is broadly divided into two types, based on histology and immunohistochemistry features: adenocarcinoma or squamous cell carcinoma.

5. All lung cancers should be tested for PD-L1. Immunohistochemistry is used for testing of PD-L1.

6. Adenocarcinoma of lung are always tested for biomarkers. On the other hand, squamous cell cancers are very unlikely to have biomarkers, so in them biomarkers are not always tested. Note that PD-L1 is tested in both adenocarcinoma and squamous cell carcinoma.

7. Biomarkers are present in only a minority of adenocarcinoma.

8. Biomarkers are markers found in cancer cells. If a biomarker is present, then it can be targeted by a specific drug which targets the biomarker itself or its products. If a biomarker is present and the drug targeting that biomarker is used, then the chances of achieving a good response are

increased, and the toxicity will also be low.

9. Following are the biomarkers tested in metastatic lung cancer:
   1. EGFR mutation
   2. ALK gene rearrangement
   3. ROS1 gene rearrangement
   4. BRAF V600E mutation
   5. MET mutation
   6. RET gene rearrangement
   7. NTRK gene fusion
   8. HER2 mutation
   9. Tumor mutation burden
10. Note that if one biomarker is present, the chances of other biomarkers being present are almost nil.
11. Some biomarkers may be tested by blood samples, this method is known as liquid biopsy.

Q13. I have metastatic lung cancer and my cancer shows the presence of overactive EGFR mutation. What is the best treatment for me?

Answer: EGFR mutation signals the cancer cells to grow, it can be blocked with targeted therapy.

If EGFR mutation is present, there are many drug

available for targeting it. Compared with chemo-therapy these drugs produce better responses and are less harmful. The options for the first line of therapy are:

1. Osimertinib
2. Afatinib
3. Dacomitinib
4. Afatinib
5. Erlotinib
6. Gefitinib

Most experts, myself included, prefer osimertinib to start with because it has been proven to halt cancer cell growth for the longest period of time. Your doctor may choose another drug.

All of these drugs are taken orally. Compared with chemotherapy, they are associated with lesser side effect but side effects are there. Main side effects are diarrhea, rash etc. These side effects are manageable with proper supportive care. Please ask your doctor about the side effects in detail.

Q14. I have been taking a targeted therapy for my EGFR mutated metastatic lung cancer. What are my chances of cure?

Answer: it is a fact that metastatic lung cancer can not be cured with presently available drugs. The aims of metastatic lung cancer treatment are to improve the quality of life, reduce the symptoms, extending life span and to prevent cancer from progressing for the longest possible time.

If you are taking an EGFR targeting drug for metastatic lung cancer, it has the potential to fulfil all of the above mentioned goals. But after some period of time, the cancer will not respond to it anymore. If this happens, it may be due to a number of reasons. One of the most common reason for the failure of an EGFR targeting drug is development of T790M mutation.

Once the metastatic lung cancer starts to progress while a patient is on an EGFR targeting drug, it is important to again assess for EGFR mutation status. If T790M mutation is found, osimertinib is the preferred drug. Osimertinib is very effective against T790M mutation.

If osimertinib was prescribed as initial therapy and the metastatic lung cancer starts to progress on it after some time, further options are very limited. Most experts advice to keep taking osimertinib coupled with symptomatic/local treatment.

If on the other hand, the initial drug was other than osimertinib and at the time of progression, T790M mutation is present; then osimertinib is the best possible choice. If at the time of progression, T790M mutation is not present then either the same drug can be continued or treatment may be started for the histologic type.

Q15. I have metastatic lung cancer and my cancer shows the presence of ALK rearrangement. What is the best treatment for me?

Answer: ALK rearrangement can be targeted with modern day medicines. These drugs produce wonderful responses and extend the life of a patient significantly more compared with chemotherapy.

There are following four drugs which are available for first line therapy of ALK rearrangement positive metastatic lung cancer:
1. Alectinib
2. Crizotinib
3. Ceretinib
4. Brigatinib

All of the these drugs are available as pills for oral intake. Please ask your doctor about their side effects and the proper way of taking these medicines, for example whether to take on an empty stomach or after eating.

Your doctor may choose any of the four approved drugs for you. Most experts recommend that alectinib is the preferred drug in all patients with ALK rearranged metastatic lung cancer, because it has shown to control cancer cell growth for the longest period of time.

Q16. I have been taking a targeted therapy for my ALK rearranged metastatic lung cancer. What are my chances of cure?

Answer: it is a fact that metastatic lung cancer can not be cured with presently available drugs. The aims of metastatic lung cancer treatment are to improve the quality of life, reduce the symptoms, extending life span and to prevent cancer from progressing for the longest possible time.

ALK targeting drugs have the potential to fulfil the above mentioned goals but it is a fact that after some time cancer progresses. Following are options for further treatment if cancer progresses on an ALK targeting drug:

1. If alectinib or ceretinib or brigatinib was the initially used drug, then there are three options for further treatment:

   1. Switching to lorlatinib. Lorlatinib is an ALK targeting drug approved for use after the metastatic lung cancer progresses on the first line of therapy.

   2. Staying on the drug that you are already taking.

   3. Starting treatment depending on the histologic type.

2. If crizotinib was the initially used drug, then there are three options for further treatment:

   1. Switching to alectinib or ceretinib or brigatinib.

      1. If the cancer progresses on any of these drugs, then switching to lorlatinib is an option.

   2. Staying on crizotinib.

   3. Starting treatment depending on the histologic type.

Q17. I have metastatic lung cancer and my cancer shows the presence of ROS1 rearrangement. What is the best treatment for me?

Answer: ROS1 rearrangement can be targeted with modern day medicines. These drugs produce wonderful responses and extend the life of a patient significantly more compared with chemotherapy.

There are following two drugs which are available for first line therapy of ROS1 rearrangement positive metastatic lung cancer:

1.   Crizotinib
2.   Ceretinib

Both of the these drugs are available as pills for oral intake. Please ask your doctor about their side effects and the proper way of taking these medicines, for example whether to take on an empty stomach or after eating.

Your doctor may choose any of the two approved drugs for you. Most experts recommend that crizotinib is the preferred drug in all patients with ROS1 rearranged metastatic lung cancer, because it has shown to control cancer cell growth for the longest period of time.

Q18. I have been taking a targeted therapy for my ROS1 rearranged metastatic lung cancer. What are my chances of cure?

Answer: it is a fact that metastatic lung cancer can not be cured with presently available drugs. The aims of metastatic lung cancer treatment are to improve the quality of life, reduce the symptoms, extending life span and to prevent cancer from progressing for the longest possible time.

ROS1 targeting drugs have the potential to fulfil the above mentioned goals but it is a fact that after some time cancer progresses. Following are options for further treatment if cancer progresses on a ROS1 targeting drug:

1. Switching to lorlatinib. Lorlatinib is an ROS1 targeting drug which is approved for treatment after failure of first line of therapy.

2. Starting treatment based on histologic type.

Q19. I have metastatic lung cancer and my cancer shows the presence of BRAF V600E mutation. What is the best treatment for me?

Answer: BRAF V600E mutation can be targeted with modern day medicines. These drugs produce wonderful responses and extend the life of a patient significantly more compared with chemotherapy.

There are following drugs which are available for first line therapy of BRAF V600E mutation positive metastatic lung cancer:
1.   Dabrafenib plus trametinib
2.   Dabrafenib
3.   Vemurafenib

Note that some experts may recommend using conventional chemotherapy in BRAF V600E mutation positive metastatic lung cancer. Please ask your doctor about the reasons of choosing this approach, if such is the case.

All of the these drugs are available as pills for oral intake. Please ask your doctor about their side effects and the proper way of taking these medicines, for example whether to take on an empty stomach or after eating.

Q20. I have been taking a targeted therapy for my BRAF V600E mutant metastatic lung cancer. What are my chances of cure?

Answer: it is a fact that metastatic lung cancer can not be cured with presently available drugs. The aims of metastatic lung cancer treatment are to improve the quality of life, reduce the symptoms, extending life span and to prevent cancer from progressing for the longest possible time.

BRAF V600E mutation targeting drugs have the potential to fulfil the above mentioned goals but it is a fact that after some time cancer progresses. Following are options for further treatment if cancer progresses on a BRAF V600E mutation targeting drug:

1.   Starting treatment based on histologic type.

Q21. I have metastatic lung cancer and my cancer shows the presence of NTRK gene fusion. What is

DR. BHRATRI BHUSHAN

the best treatment for me?

Answer: NTRK gene fusion can be targeted with modern day medicines. These drugs produce wonderful responses and extend the life of a patient significantly more compared with chemotherapy.

Larotrectinib is available for first line therapy of NTRK gene fusion positive metastatic lung cancer.

Note that some experts may recommend using conventional chemotherapy in NTRK gene fusion positive metastatic lung cancer. Please ask your doctor about the reasons of choosing this approach, if such is the case.

This drug is available as pills for oral intake. Please ask your doctor about its side effects and the proper way of taking it, for example whether to take on an empty stomach or after eating.

Q22. I have been taking a targeted therapy for my NTRK gene fusion metastatic lung cancer. What are my chances of cure?

Answer: it is a fact that metastatic lung cancer can not be cured with presently available drugs. The aims of metastatic lung cancer treatment are to improve the quality of life, reduce the symptoms, extending life span and to prevent cancer from progressing for the longest possible time.

NTRK gene fusion targeting drugs have the potential to fulfil the above mentioned goals but it is a fact that after some time cancer progresses. Following are options for further treatment if cancer progresses on a NTRK gene fusion targeting drug:

1. Starting treatment based on histologic type.

Q23. I have metastatic lung cancer and my cancer shows the presence of PD-L1. What is the best treatment for me?

Answer: please remember these points:

1. PD-L1 is tested in all patients with metastatic lung cancer.
2. PD-L1 results are expressed as percent values.
3. If you have targetable mutations, then PD-L1 directed therapy is **not** used as first line because of very low response

rates with PD-L1 directed therapy in such cases.

4. The drugs which target, PD-1/PD-L1 or CTLA4 are called immune checkpoint inhibitors. They are colloquially called immunotherapy.

5. Remember that immunotherapy also has many side effects.

6. Remember that immunotherapy doesn't guarantee cure.

The choice of therapy depends on the histology of metastatic lung cancer and the % value of PD-L1.

Following are the options for first line therapy of metastatic "adenocarcinoma" lung, as well as large cell lung cancer and unknown types:

1. If PD-L1 is 50% or more, pembrolizumab is the preferred option.

2. If PD-L1 is 1-49% the combination of cisplatin (or carboplatin) plus pemetrexed plus pembrolizumab is preferred.

3. Carboplatin plus paclitaxel plus bevacizumab plus atezolizumab is also an option.

Following are the options for first line therapy of metastatic "squamous cell carcinoma" lung:
1. If PD-L1 is 50% or more, pembrolizumab is the preferred option.
2. If PD-L1 is 1-49% the combination of cisplatin (or carboplatin) plus paclitaxel plus pembrolizumab is preferred.

Please understand that if targetable mutation is present, the above mentioned therapies are not preferred. For example, if a patient with metastatic lung cancer has ALK rearrangement and also has PD-L1 more than 50%, then he will be treated with an ALK mutation targeting drug (not immunotherapy). Immunotherapy is the preferred option in patients with metastatic lung cancer who **don't** have any targetable mutation.

Q24. Are there side effects of immunotherapy?

Answer: immunotherapy in lung cancer is in the form of immune checkpoint inhibitors (ICIs). These drugs act on immune "checkpoints" and lift the blocks that tumor cells form to deceive a patient's immune system. Once these blocks are lifted, the immune system of the patient attacks the cancer cells. So, in a way, immunotherapy drugs harness the power of the patient's own immune system.

The immune checkpoint inhibitor drugs are available for administration as intravenous injections. They are usually given once every 2, 3 or 4 weeks, depending on the protocol being used.

The side effects that are commonly seen with chemotherapy are not so commonly seen with immunotherapy. That being said, there are many side effects of immunotherapy. Many of these side effects occur due to the activation of immune system, which harms the organs of the body. The side effects will manifest according to the affected organ(s). Please ask your doctor about the side effects of immunotherapy, their prevention and management.

Q25. I have metastatic lung cancer, without any targetable mutation. I was started on chemotherpy plus immunotherapy and now my cancer has progressed. What is the best option for me now?

Answer: in question number 23 we have discussed about the first line therapy for metastatic lung cancer that doesn't have any targetable mutation. Such patients may be started on chemotherapy plus immunotherapy combinations, as we have discussed or they may be started on immunotherapy alone or chemotherapy alone. After some time, the cancer progresses on the first line therapy.

Once the cancer progresses, second line therapy is started. Following are options for second line therapy in patients with metastatic lung cancer without any targetable mutation:

1.   Pembrolizumab
2.   Nivolumab
3.   Atezolizumab
4.   Chemotherpy
5.   Ramucirumab plus chemotherapy

There may be some patients who will not be able to tolerate any therapy due to their poor performance status. If such is the case, then only supportive care is continued and cancer directed therapy is not used.

Q26. I am suffering from metastatic lung cancer. My cancer doesn't have any targetable mutations and due to some reason, I will not be able to take immunotherapy. What is the best treatment for me?

Answer: there may be a number of reasons which may make a patient unfit for receiving immunotherapy. If that's the case then chemotherpy is the only option, if the performance status permits. Chemotherapy is usually started as soon as the diagnosis is made. Chemotherapy is given in "cycles", depending on the drugs being used. Usually a combination of drugs is used, which is known as "doublet" chemotherapy. This doublet chemotherapy is continued for 4 to 6 cycles.

After the completion of 4 to 6 cycles, one of the following is done:

1.   One of the two drugs may be continued indefinitely, until disease progression on unacceptable toxicity. It is known as continuation maintenance.
2.   A different drug than the two being used initially may be continued indefinitely, until disease progression or unacceptable toxicity. It is known as switch maintenance.
3.   All treatment is stopped and the patients is put under surveillance.

Chemotherapy is toxic and its side effects range from mild to life threatening. Many precautions are taken beforehand to reduce the intensity and frequency of side effects. Please ask your doctor in detail about the side effects, their prevention and management.

Q27. What is the best treatment for metastatic small cell lung cancer?

Answer: as we have already discussed, lung cancer is basically of two types: small cell and non small cell.

The treatment of small cell lung cancer is very different from non small cell lung cancer.

Small cell lung cancer is not tested for targetable mutations. It is treated with chemotherapy. Immunotherapy is used in combination with chemotherapy in certain situations.

The chemotherpy of choice for metastatic small cell lung cancer is a combination of a platinum drug with etoposide.

Some patients with small cell lung cancer may need to receive prophylactic radiation therapy to the brain and possibly to lungs. Please ask your doctor in detail about the treatment options.

Q29. I am suffering from stage IV lung cancer. What are my chances of cure?

Answer: as we have discussed, stage IV lung cancer is not a single disease entity. The treatment as well as prognosis of stage IV lung cancer subsets are different.

It is out of the scope of this book to discuss the details of prognostic factors and their interplay. I will provide you salient points to build some basic knowledge regarding prognosis of metastatic lung cancer:

1. Metastatic lung cancer is not considered curable with currently available therapies.
2. However, extraordinary progress has been made in extending the life of patients.
3. The prognosis depends on many factors, for example:
    1. Overall medical fitness of the patient. It is often expressed as performance status.

2. Presence of other diseases.
3. Histologic type of cancer.
4. Presence or absence of targetable mutations.

4. Now we will explore some clinical situations:

    1. If targetable mutations are present, the prognosis is better. For instance, if ALK rearrangement is present, then with ALK targeting drugs, a patient can be expected to survive for upto 4 years or more.
    2. If targetable mutations are absent, then immunotherapy based treatment is the preferred choice. The prognosis is not as good.
    3. With use of only chemotherapy, the overall survival is expected to be less than one year.
    4. If brain metastases are present and targetable mutations are not present, then survival is expected to be less than 6 months.

These are broad generalisations. Every patient is different. I have many patients, who are receiving only chemotherapy in form of maintenance and are surviving after 5 years. It all depends on how your cancer will respond to therapies.

I must request you to keep asking your doctor to provide you the best of palliative and supportive care. It has been found in studies that timely use of palliative care improves not just the quality of life, but also overall survival.

Medicines and data are one thing, but the most important part of the treatment is your willpower. Stay positive and keep yourself informed. I wish you and your loved ones the best of health. It will be my honour and privilege to support you in any way. In case of any queries, please contact me at bhratri@gmail.com

Printed in Great Britain
by Amazon